Alkaline Diet

A Comprehensive Manual On Effortless Recipes Designed
To Restore Ph Balance And Boost The Body's Innate
Healing Mechanisms

*(Effortless And Straightforward Smoothie Recipes For
Alkalizing Your Body, Abundantly Enriched With
Essential Nutrients)*

Samuel Cheung

TABLE OF CONTENT

In Order To Uphold An Alkaline Milieu Within The Body, Magnesium Is Just As Crucial As Calcium.

In the case of young individuals, x-rays do not ascertain the presence of bone erosion resulting from insufficient calcium levels. In advanced age, there is a reduction in bone density as a result of calcium depletion caused by the elimination of acid burden, which allows us to perceive the deterioration in the bones.

In the younger demographic, the level of acid load is comparatively minimal, thereby enabling the blood to utilize alternative substances like bicarbonate for the purpose of eliminating this load. In younger individuals, the extraction of calcium from the skeletal structure serves as the body's ultimate measure for eliminating acidic waste. Acidification is a protracted and gradual phenomenon, with its consequences becoming apparent solely over time. Osteoporosis primarily manifests in advanced age due to the body's diminished ability to effectively eliminate acid load through the mechanisms employed during youth. The elderly individuals are required to utilize the calcium and magnesium stored within their bones. In order to prevent osteoporosis, it is necessary to refrain from consuming acidic food and beverages and instead incorporate foods that are abundant in calcium and magnesium into our diet. For instance, our physical systems necessitate the consumption of 32 servings of water and a substantial intake of calcium derived from our skeletal structure to counteract the acidic burden imposed by a mere serving of carbonated cola. We consume a daily dosage of 50 mg of calcium to counterbalance the acidic load. You might perceive this as being inconsequential. Nevertheless, the gradual process of acidification over the course of several years results in the extraction of minerals from the bones, ultimately accumulating up to a staggering 400,000 mg. This quantity is tantamount to depleting half of the calcium content in a woman's bones and one-third in the case of men. This implies that, on average, women experience a 50% reduction in bone density during old age, whereas men encounter a 33% decline.

Chronic acidification is the underlying cause of osteoporosis.

Acidification contributes to the occurrence of various other ailments.

It is widely acknowledged that the consumption of acid is responsible for dental decay. Tooth decay is prevalent among children who consume excessive quantities of sweets due to the acidification triggered by sugar consumption. The presence of acidity, in conjunction with the presence of sugar, facilitates the proliferation of bacteria. In addition, this induces the development of periodontal disease.

The oral cavity typically exhibits an alkaline nature. The process of carbohydrate digestion initiates in the oral cavity through the action of an enzyme known as amylase. Amylase is retained within the saliva and exclusively operates within alkaline environments. Heightened acidification within the human body leads to a corresponding escalation in saliva acidity. Consequently, the proper functioning of amylase is impaired, consequently hindering the proper digestion of sugar and carbohydrates. Poor digestion contributes to the acidification occurring in the oral cavity.

Iodine is a mineral that exhibits optimal performance in alkaline conditions. The utilization of iodine may be impaired as a result of excessive acidification, potentially leading to a reduction in thyroid function. A decrement in thyroid function results in hypothyroidism, wherein one may experience a propensity for weight gain.

The primary protein present in the human body is collagen. Acidification hardens collagen. The presence of collagen in our joints and skin leads to a loss of flexibility and elasticity due to its process of hardening. The integumentary system undergoes the formation of wrinkles and experiences dehydration. The process of acidification exerts a significant impact on the aging of the skin.

In an acidic milieu, there is a reduction in the availability of oxygen to the blood and tissues. This facilitates the production of anaerobic bacteria and augments the proclivity towards infections.

Bacterial and fungal infections manifest with greater frequency.

The efficacy of intercellular communication relies upon the pliancy of the cellular membrane. Acidification hardens cell membranes. Hardened membranes impede cellular communication, particularly within the cerebral region.

Moreover, acidification has an impact on conditions such as insomnia, depression, and memory impairment. The hormone melatonin is essential for facilitating a restful sleep during the night. The human body synthesizes serotonin as a means of mitigating or alleviating symptoms of depression. The formation of memories is contingent upon effective inter-neuronal communication within our complex nervous system. The acidification process hampers intercellular communication crucial for the functioning of melatonin, serotonin, and neurons.

To elucidate further: As previously stated, the primary objective of chemical reactions within cells is the generation of energy. The energy is generated through the combustion of glucose derived from ingested food and oxygen within the cellular environment. Similar to how the residual product of burning is ash, the generation of energy within our cells results in the production of acidic waste. Each individual cell produces acidic waste on a continuous basis. Every cell possesses the capacity to undertake a partial removal of this acid. When an excessive amount of acid is present, it initiates an assault on the cell membrane, targeting it as the most susceptible site. This leads to the acidification of the cellular membrane and consequently, the hardening and diminished sensitivity of the said membrane.

Consequently, this creates a challenging situation wherein cells encounter difficulty in adhering to hormonal directives, thereby resulting in insomnia, chronic fatigue, and depression.

Insulin is an additional hormone which transmits directives to the cellular structures. Insulin functions akin to a key, facilitating the unlocking of a molecular receptor situated within the cell membrane. The key serves as an access point for the glucose transporter protein GLUT4, enabling the facilitation of glucose influx into the cell. The inability to access insulin renders the door inoperable, thereby preventing the entry of glucose. Once the cell membrane undergoes stiffening, the lock becomes non-functional. The quantity of insulin present in the bloodstream is inadequate to facilitate the opening of this door, consequently compelling the pancreas to generate additional insulin. However, due to the process of acidification, the additional amount of insulin proves to be insufficient as the doorway in the membrane develops resistance. This condition is referred to as insulin resistance.

Chapter Five: Examination of pH Levels

In preceding chapters, you acquired extensive knowledge regarding alkalinity and acidity. You have acquired knowledge on the appropriate dietary choices and principles governing the alkaline diet. Therefore, how can one determine if their endeavors are yielding desirable results? This can be accomplished through the process of pH testing.

It is recommended to perform pH testing on a daily basis. It is a cost-effective undertaking that can be completed efficiently and effortlessly. In fact, conducting the test on a weekly basis is adequate. In the end, the frequency at which you choose to engage in this activity is at your discretion. During the initial month of your dietary regimen, adhering to a daily routine is highly recommended to enable accurate assessment of the extent to which your choices are contributing to your progress. This not only guarantees that you remain focused but also observing the transformations can serve as a catalyst to maintain your motivation.

When conducting pH tests in a residential setting, it is customary to employ saliva or urine samples as a means of measurement. It is desirable for your results to fall within the range of 7.2 to 7.4, signifying the efficacy of your dietary plan, adherence to it, and the consequent advantages derived from your alkaline diet.

At drugstores, you can procure strips specifically designed for performing this test. Kindly adhere to the provided guidelines to ensure the attainment of reliable outcomes. Primarily, you shall be responsible for applying the necessary volume of urine or saliva onto the testing strip. This action will initialize the strip and provide you with a numerical identifier. Merely document your values in order to monitor your pH levels.

Prior to conducting the examination, it is advised to be conscientious of your actions during the preceding 60 minutes. As an illustration, in the event that one were to consume a significantly alkaline substance, it could serve as an indicator of the urine possessing a higher alkaline level. Due to this circumstance, it is necessary to refrain from consuming beverages with a high alkaline content within a 60-minute period before conducting the test. Refrain from consuming highly alkaline food items or using dental hygiene products that consist of baking soda within a span of 60 minutes prior to the test, using your saliva. This measure will serve to avert the occurrence of an erroneous outcome.

The optimal time for testing is at the onset of the day. Please ensure that you complete the task immediately upon waking up. When using the saliva strips, it is customary to place them within the oral cavity, specifically in proximity to the inner cheeks. Retain it for the duration specified by the instructions. During this particular period of the day, it is expected that the pH level of your saliva falls within the range of 6.8 to 7.2. It is important to note that the results may take up to a minute to become apparent, dependent on the specific test kit employed.

Following the analysis of your saliva sample, please proceed to obtain your urine testing kit. This task should be prioritized at the commencement of the day. To collect a fresh urine sample, it is recommended to delicately position the stick within the flow of your urine. The optimal pH range should fall approximately between 6.8 and 7.2. It is advisable to allow at least one minute for accurate reading, thus ensuring that the strip delivers the finalized result.

In the event that the pH level of either your urine or saliva falls below 6.8, it signifies an elevated degree of acidity. Please ensure that you closely monitor your dietary intake and adequately hydrate yourself to promote the restoration of optimal alkalinity. Additionally, it is suggested by some experts to conduct testing on the second urine sample of the day. Simply adhere to the identical procedure for this particular task. Merely repeat the action during your second occurrence of morning urination. There should be a minimum gap of one hour following your initial test before consuming any food. You are permitted to consume water during the interval between the two examinations.

High Acid Foods

Vegetables: None!

Fruit Varieties: Blueberries, cranberries, strawberries, raspberries; Juices sweetened with fruit extract.

Meat and fish options consist of beef, pork, cultivated fish, shellfish, and various preparations of eggs such as poached, fried, and scrambled.

Additional items include alcoholic beverages, coffee, cocoa, black tea, preserves, honey, vinegar, soy sauce, yeast, mustard, cheese, as well as artificial sweeteners and syrups.

Next, we shall examine alkaline foods. Below is a compilation of foods that exhibit varying levels of alkalinity, categorized as mildly, moderately, and highly alkaline:

Mildly Alkaline Foods

The following vegetables are: cauliflower, Brussels sprouts, artichokes, carrots, chives, zucchini, rhubarb, leeks, peas, watercress, mushrooms, and tomatoes.

The fruit options include avocado, grapefruit, coconut, oranges, bananas, and cherries.

Dairy products available include goat milk and goat cheese, whey, soy-based cheese, and almond milk.

Alternative: The following items are also available: quinoa, lentils, legumes, flaxseed oil, avocado oil, ginger infusion, canola oil, chestnuts, wild rice, unrefined sugar, and pure honey.

Moderately alkaline

Assorted vegetables: Including capsicum (peppers), ginger, beetroot, cabbage, celery, radish, okra, and red onion.

Fruits: Lemons, limes, kiwis, pears, and apples.

Additional options include rice syrup, maple syrup, almonds, butter beans, and white beans.

Highly Alkaline Foods

These are the various types of vegetables included: cucumber, kelp, kale, grasses, sprouted beans, alfalfa sprouts, broccoli, garlic, and seaweed.

Selection of fruits: watermelon, cantaloupe, passion fruit, and raisins.

Other options include: green tea, herbal tea, Himalayan salt, alkaline water, agar agar (natural gelatine substitute), walnuts, and lemon-infused water.

Strategies for Integrating Foods to Attain Optimal Nutritional Harmony
The nutrients contained in the food we consume undergo the processes of digestion, absorption, and eventually metabolism, resulting in the production of acidic or alkaline substances that enter the bloodstream. It is crucial to incorporate alkaline foods alongside acidic foods in one's diet to attain a state of longevity, robust health, and overall well-being. The conventional dietary patterns observed in Australia are characterized by an excessive consumption of high-fat meats and heavily processed foods, while inadequately incorporating a sufficient quantity of vegetables and

fruits to counterbalance their acidic impact.

The issue does not primarily stem from a specific food item, but rather from the imperative of ensuring that one's diet comprises a balanced mix of acidic and alkaline foods. What measures can be taken to mitigate the adverse effects of internal acid accumulation resulting from misguided dietary selections?

Presented herewith are a selection of beneficial recommendations and insights pertaining to the pairing of food items:

It is imperative to take into consideration that the ensuing regulations solely pertain to concentrated forms of proteins, carbohydrates, and fats.

1. Refrain from the amalgamation of carbohydrates and acidic food components.

As an illustration, the consumption of berries in conjunction with bread, rice, or potatoes has the capacity to inhibit the function of the enzyme 'ptyalin,' which plays a crucial role in the breakdown of carbohydrates within the digestive system. The acetic acid present in vinegar, for instance, disrupts the process of salivary digestion. If it suits your preference, consider consuming fruits with acidic properties approximately 40 minutes prior to a meal.

2. Tomatoes and starchy foods are not a compatible combination.
Tomatoes possess three types of acids, namely, oxalic, citric, and malic acids, which are present in tomatoes and their concentration becomes more concentrated through the process of cooking. These acids inhibit the enzymatic breakdown of starches in the oral cavity. It would be more prudent to juxtapose tomatoes with verdant, foliated vegetables instead.
Individuals afflicted with hyperacidity ought to refrain from consuming food combinations that

consist of both acidic and starchy elements. It initiates the process of fermentation and elevates the levels of acidity within the body.

3. It is recommended to refrain from consuming a combination of concentrated carbohydrates and concentrated proteins.

The rationale for exercising caution stems from the disparate physiological mechanisms of digestion at play. Gastric digestion is fundamentally different from salivary digestion, and it is not possible for these processes to occur simultaneously. The gastric acids halt the process of salivary digestion, leading to the initiation of fermentation.

In essence, the process of protein digestion gives rise to concentrated gastric juices that impede the digestion of starch.

To the greatest extent feasible, it is advisable to refrain from consuming cheese, meat, eggs, nuts, and similar items concurrently with bread, potatoes, cereals, and related food items.

4. It is advised against including two concentrated proteins in meals.
It is advisable to consume a single variety of protein during each meal. Consuming multiple concentrated proteins leads to the secretion of gastric juices that vary in nature, type, and intensity. Frequently, the combination of such diverse juices tends to be incompatible.
Refrain from consuming nuts and cheese, or eggs and milk, or other compatible food combinations, within the same meal.

5. The combination of concentrated proteins and fats is not compatible
When lipids are metabolized, they undergo conversion into fatty acids. Fatty acids have been found to impede the synthesis of gastric secretions such as pepsin and hydrochloric acid. Additionally, it

inhibits the necessary digestive process for proteins while also halting the function of gastric glands. It is advisable to abstain from consuming nuts, cheese, eggs, and other such items in conjunction with butter, oil, and cream.

6. It is not recommended to mix acid-fruits with concentrated proteins.
Citrus fruits, such as oranges, along with berries and pineapples, should not be ingested in conjunction with meat or eggs (though they do not hinder the digestion of cheeses and nuts).
The acids present in acidic fruits have the effect of retarding the process of protein digestion, consequently contributing to the occurrence of putrefaction, which refers to the decay of organic matter. It is advisable to refrain from consuming fruit juices in conjunction with eggs or meat.

7. Love sweets? Do not consume them alongside starchy substances.

If one possesses an inclination for sugary indulgence, it is advisable to refrain from consuming preserves, confections, nectar, and likewise in conjunction with bread, potatoes, cereal, and similar fare. The phenomenon that occurs is the deception of the taste buds by the presence of a sweet flavor. The oral cavity generates salivary secretions (which lack ptyalin enzyme essential for the digestion of starch) while facilitating the breakdown of sugars.

However, the starch remains undigested, leading to subsequent fermentation. This holds particular significance in the context of desserts, particularly those which involve the use of starches, such as cakes, cleverly concealed with a sugary layer on top, such as a syrup glaze.

8. Consume sugary fruits and acidic fruits separately.

While fruits are a nutritious means of promoting overall well-being, it is advisable to consume sweet fruits and acidic fruits separately. The sugars derived from acidic fruits, such as pineapples, undergo digestion within approximately one hour. Nevertheless, the sugars derived from sweet fruits such as figs, raisins, grapes, and cherries necessitate a digestion period of approximately three hours.

It is advisable to avoid combining them, as the metabolic breakdown of sweet-sugars can disrupt the digestion process of acid-sugars. Consequently, the sugars derived from the acidic fruits will undergo fermentation as a consequence of slowed digestive processes.

9. Enjoy eating Juicy Melons? Eat them alone!

The majority of melon varieties, such as watermelon, muskmelon, casaba melon, cantaloupes, and honeydew melons, undergo rapid digestion within the stomach. Therefore, it is preferable to consume them in solitude. Ingesting them alongside other food items often leads to a sensation of weightiness and unease. They require exclusive use of the stomach for a brief duration.

10. Consume milk in isolation without simultaneous intake of food. Milk undergoes digestion primarily within the duodenum, a section of the small intestine, as opposed to the stomach. Moreover, milk cream inhibits the secretion of gastric juices in the stomach for some time after consumption. Therefore, it is advisable to consume milk in isolation and allow for a period of digestion prior to consuming any other food.

Compendium of Moderately to Incredibly Alkaline Food Items and Their Utilization Techniques

There exists a variety of levels of alkaline foods. The items mentioned in this list are widely recognized as being among the finest, and it is advisable to strive for a minimum attainment of 80% in consuming a mixture of foods that range from highly alkaline to moderately alkaline. This approach will serve as a catalyst for initiating your desired lifestyle transformation.

Select these food items and incorporate them into your dietary intake:

Avocados are an excellent dietary option for replacing most animal-based fats due to their rich content of natural fats.

✓ Broccoli is renowned for its superior alkalinity properties, making it an exceptional choice for maintaining optimal pH levels in the body. Consume alongside a variety of leafy vegetables and low-fat sources of protein in order to counteract the production of intestinal gas.

Cabbage, in virtually all its variations, possesses notable purifying properties.

Consuming an adequate amount of celery, either through ingestion or by extracting its juice, has the potential to mitigate hypertension.

Cucumber offers numerous health benefits and enhances the flavor of salads.

Moreover, garlic serves as an exceptional antibacterial agent.

✓ Green vegetables and sprouts - such as alfalfa, wheatgrass, kale, and spinach - that are effortlessly suitable for juicing.

Parsley can be effectively incorporated into juice as well.

✓ Tomato – consume as is in sliced form. Additionally, it has the capacity to inhibit the development of prostate cancer.

Now, let us consider foods that have a slightly to moderately alkaline pH:

✓ Artichokes - delectable when prepared with a modest quantity of organic butter and a hint of Himalayan sea salt, which is also alkaline in nature.

✓ Asparagus – an aesthetically unique vegetable that boasts a wealth of nutritional benefits.

✓ Brussels sprouts – delectable and rich in beneficial nutrients.

✔ Beets - rich in nutrients.

Cauliflower bears resemblance to broccoli, albeit with a more pronounced flavor.

Leeks, in all their varieties, exhibit excellent compatibility with stir frying.

✓ Baby Potatoes – it may be difficult to comprehend, but it is worth noting that the majority of potatoes exhibit alkaline properties. These are too.

Snap peas are the optimal choice when it comes to selecting peas.

✔ Pumpkin is exquisite when stewed or consumed cooked,

complemented by a sprinkle of Himalayan sea salt.

✓ Onion – beneficial for gastrointestinal health.

Squash in all its varieties is acceptable.

By incorporating exclusively organic variants of these foods into your diet in their natural, unprocessed form, you will transition from a condition of excessive acidity to a gradual improvement in alkaline levels (it is worth noting that higher values in this context are more desirable, although we will refer to this as a decrease in acidity).

Now that you have been informed of the most optimal alkaline foods, it is important to bear in mind that there exist numerous alternative alkaline foods and beverages. Therefore, we encourage you to persist in your search for additional food options that can be incorporated into your diet.

Diversity enhances one's existence and supports the maintenance of a balanced dietary regimen.

Additional Food Items to Take into Consideration

There exist several additional food items and beverages that could potentially be included in your dietary regimen, with particular emphasis on teas. Additionally, it is prudent to contemplate the inclusion of various culinary options and associated dietary suggestions indicated herein as supplementary accompaniments or feasible substitutes which possess, at the very least, a moderate alkaline nature.

Consider transitioning from coffee to whole leaf teas as an alternate beverage selection. This encompassing choice encompasses teas such as green, peppermint, lavender, yerba mate, rooibos or bush tea, ginger, and turmeric tea, all of which are esteemed for their alkaline properties. Ensure that you exclusively utilize intact leaf and unrefined teas.

✓ Viable alkaline condiments – edibles such as chives, basil, peppers, red onions, chia seeds, hemp seeds, sesame seeds, numerous herbs and spices that are already present in your collection of seasonings.

✓ The blood grouping diet has been formulated as a result of extensive research conducted by Dr. DaDamo over the course of several years. His book "Eat Right for Your Type," which has achieved bestseller status on the New York Times list, has enjoyed enduring popularity for years. This comprehensive work encompasses extensive research, compelling case studies, and a thorough analysis of the underlying causes of our ailments. I would suggest that you consider incorporating his book into your library in order to encompass information that falls outside the purview of this manual:

Incorporate these ultimate recommendations to complement your comprehensive understanding of genuine health and wellness and the methods to attain it.

The Guidelines And Prohibitions Of The Alkaline Diet

While the initial chapter comprehensively covered the fundamental knowledge necessary for embarking on the Alkaline Diet journey, this subsequent chapter will primarily underscore the permissible and prohibited food items. You will also acquire knowledge regarding prevalent misconceptions linked to the Alkaline Diet.

To commence, let us thoroughly examine a comprehensive inventory of nutrition items permissible for consumption within the Alkaline Diet.

Prescribed Food Items and Nutritional Approaches

Fruits and Vegetables

It is advisable to opt for fresh vegetables and fruits whenever feasible, as they have a tendency to contribute to an elevation in the alkalinity of the body. When juxtaposed with all other food compounds, they emerge as the most optimal source of alkalinity for maintaining blood pH levels. There are several delectable and captivating ones that you should be attentive to. These include:

Mushroom

Dates

Watermelon

Raisins

Ripe bananas

Spinach

Ginger

Grapefruit

Citrus

Tomatoes

Avocados

Summer Black Radish

Red beet

Almonds

Alfalfa Grass

Celery

Kale

Oregano

Cucumber

Cabbage

Jicama

Endive

Garlic

Wheat Grass

Figs

Green beans

Broccoli

Eat Raw Food

It is crucial to acknowledge that one should consistently endeavor to consume their food in its raw state. It should be noted that the aforementioned statement is not intended as an endorsement of consuming raw meat in a manner similar to that of hyenas. However, it is evident that opting for uncooked vegetables and fruits, whenever feasible, is preferable due to their classification as "Biogenic."

When engaged in the process of cooking, the essential minerals with alkalizing properties become depleted from the food. Therefore, endeavor to enhance your intake of uncooked fruits and vegetables by means such as extracting their juices or gently subjecting them to steam for optimal outcomes.

Embrace Plant-Based Proteins

It would be advisable for you to consider incorporating plant-based proteins into your diet. "Optimal selections comprise

Steamed vegetables

Almonds

Lima beans

Navy beans

Promoting the Benefits of Alkaline Water

Alkaline waters typically exhibit a pH level ranging between 9 and 11. They are available in pre-packaged containers, but as a viable option, you may also consider opting for distilled water. It is crucial that you acknowledge the fact that water subjected to the prevailing method of filtration known as "Reverse Osmosis" has a tendency to possess a slightly acidic nature. Therefore, if your goal is to achieve alkalinity, it would be more advisable to opt for the previously mentioned bottled water or tap water. If feasible, it is recommended to consider incorporating a small quantity of baking soda or lemon juice in order to augment the alkaline properties.

Going Green

It is expected that you have attained knowledge regarding the strict prohibition of soft drinks and carbonated beverages in relation to adhering to an alkaline diet. Whenever you experience a genuine longing for a carbonated beverage, it is advisable to opt for beverages that are derived from botanical sources such as grasses or green vegetables.

If it is feasible, you may also consider seeking them in a powdered form, as they are rich in alkaline-inducing chlorophyll. Please bear in mind that chlorophyll possesses a remarkably analogous structure to that of human blood, thereby profoundly augmenting the alkalinity of the blood.

Good enough so far?

If one is truly committed, it is highly advisable to refrain from consuming the subsequent foods and engaging in the mentioned habits. They will consequently elevate the acidity levels within your body.

Chapter 2 Indicators of Excessive Acidity Levels in the Body

Below are indications that may suggest excessive acidity in the body, signaling the need for proactive measures to promote a healthier lifestyle.

One of the notable indications that your body is excessively acidic is the onset of fatigue, despite having consistently obtained a minimum of 8 hours of rest each night. Individuals with elevated levels of acidity in their physiological system often experience feelings of fatigue and diminished energy levels, even following sufficient periods of rest.

Elevated levels of acidity in the body tend to induce persistent feelings of melancholy and despondency.

Individuals who experience elevated levels of acidity in their body also exhibit a tendency to become inexplicably irritable and are prone to quick bursts of anger.

An additional indication of elevated acidic levels is the lack of ability to concentrate effectively on one's task.

Diminished immune function and increased vulnerability to viral infections, such as the common cold and influenza, is another prevalent indication of elevated acidity.

Individuals experiencing dermatological issues and dryness in their skin may have an elevated acidity level.

An indication of your body's acidity can also manifest in the form of hormonal imbalances.

Digestive concerns such as gastrointestinal disturbances, irregular bowel movements, and imbalances may arise as a result of heightened acidity within the body.

Dyspnea, chronic discomfort, dental and gingival hypersensitivity, and cervical stiffness are additional prevailing indications of systemic acidosis.

Below are additional indicators that your physiological state may exhibit excessive acidity:

Allergies

Urinary tract infections involving the bladder and kidneys.

Cardiovascular damage

Chest pain

Chronic fatigue

Diabetes

Immune deficiency

Articular discomfort and soreness in musculature.

Reduced mental clarity

Conducting a Personal pH Assessment

Measuring one's own pH can be accomplished easily by procuring a pack of pH strips through online retailers or local pharmaceutical establishments. It is advisable to conduct this test as an initial task in the morning. The acidity levels of your body will be higher if you measure it earlier, and it is advisable to refrain from consuming any food or beverage prior to conducting your initial morning examination.

Should you so desire, you have the option to conduct self-assessments both in the morning and evening. Nevertheless, exercise caution in not allowing yourself to become fixated on your pH measurements, akin to the manner in which certain individuals obsess over their own weight. The objective is to attain good health rather than striving for an ideal numerical measure. The objective is to ensure that the pH level in the morning falls within the range of 6.5 to 7.5.

The crucial aspect is that you:

Conduct examinations at consistent daily intervals

Document your discoveries in a formal written record such as a journal or notebook.

Valuable recommendations for enhancing reading precision

For saliva

Please ensure a minimum waiting period of 2 hours subsequent to consuming a meal before conducting a measurement of your salivary pH. Mouth your oral cavity with salivary secretions before proceeding to ingest them. Please perform this step once more to ensure the cleanliness and absence of acid-producing bacteria in your saliva. Please apply a small amount of saliva onto the pH strip for testing purposes. Refrain from employing water or any other fluids for the purpose of rinsing your oral cavity.

For urine

Please allow for urination to occur prior to the collection of a specimen for testing purposes. This guarantees a higher level of precision in the measurement.

To obtain an accurate reading, it is recommended to conduct the test either one hour prior to a meal or two hours post-consumption.

Chapter 3: The Beneficial Effects of the Alkaline Diet

In order for the body to adequately uphold its subtle alkaline equilibrium, it necessitates an ample provision of minerals that promote alkalinity. Furthermore, it is imperative to consume food items that do not excessively burden the body's inherent capacity to neutralize and eliminate acidic substances.

The Alkaline Diet operates through two primary mechanisms:

It excludes foods that induce acidification within the body.

It contributes essential nutrients that facilitate the process of bodily repair.

The Advantages of Adhering to an Alkaline Diet

"Presented below are a number of substantiated advantages associated with maintaining an alkaline state:

Safeguards bone density and muscle mass: Adequate intake of vitamin D and essential minerals such as magnesium, calcium, and phosphate is crucial for the development of robust bones and preservation of skeletal integrity. Alkaline diets offer robust protection to the skeletal system through the abundant provision of essential vitamins and minerals, which not only safeguard the integrity of bones but also facilitate the development of lean muscle mass. Additionally, scholarly studies have indicated that alkaline diets have been connected with an elevation in the production of growth hormone. This hormone plays a pivotal role in the development of lean muscle mass and facilitates the absorption of vitamin D, a critical component in maintaining optimal bone health and preventing bone degeneration in older individuals.

Reduces the likelihood of hypertension and stroke: The alkaline diet enhances the equilibrium between potassium and sodium, thereby safeguarding the functionality of the neurological system and the cardiovascular system. According to research findings, enhancing this ratio has been demonstrated to reduce the likelihood of experiencing hypertension and stroke.

Reduces inflammation: Nearly all modern diseases afflicting the human population stem from an underlying issue of inflammation. This can be attributed to the fact that the contemporary Western diet consists of a plethora of food items, oils, and toxins that engender this outcome. Industrial seed oils such as sunflower, soybean, canola, and corn oils, along with trans fats, refined carbohydrates, sugar, alcohol, and processed meats, can be regarded as particularly egregious examples. Each of these food items possesses a significant pro-inflammatory potential. The alkaline diet aids in the reduction of inflammation across the body through the elimination of all food items and substances that provoke inflammation from your dietary intake. In order to achieve the detoxification, healing, and promotion of a lifelong state of health, disease prevention should be prioritized over disease promotion.

Alleviates chronic pain: Research has further highlighted that consumption of an acidic diet has been linked to heightened pain levels. A study conducted by researchers has yielded the finding that the process of alkalizing the human body has the potential to alleviate the symptoms of chronic back pain.

Aids in maintaining a healthy weight: The alkaline diet contributes to the reduction of leptin levels within the body. Leptin is the satiety hormone that frequently leads to excessive food consumption when it is present in excess. In addition, the alkaline diet confers significant health benefits, providing an adequate supply of minerals that can help prevent inflammation, while also supplying vital nutrients to support the liver's ability to eliminate surplus fat-storing hormones such as cortisol from the body. The diet advocates for a highly slender physique.

Assists in promoting cancer cell apoptosis: Supporters of the alkaline diet also hold a firm belief in the diet's potential to prevent cancer. The proliferation of cancer is facilitated in a body that harbors an abundance of acidic toxins, whereas the presence of a purified, alkaline environment greatly inhibits the development of nearly all diseases.

You obtain luminous skin: The alkaline diet boasts a plethora of vitamins, antioxidants, and minerals, which serve to reinforce the health and appearance of your skin. The diet provides nourishment to the mitochondria of your fibroblasts, thereby stimulating the production of fresh reserves of collagen and elastin. The ample provision of essential minerals and vitamins contributes to the maintenance of a luminescent, radiant, and rejuvenated complexion.

Alleviates kidney complications: The alkaline diet offers significant support for optimal kidney health. Medical professionals frequently advise patients with kidney disease or individuals undergoing dialysis to adhere to the alkaline diet. The alkaline diet is highly effective in providing prevention against the formation of kidney stones.

Selecting an Appropriate Alkaline Nutrition Plan

Constructing a prosperous alkaline diet necessitates the ingestion of appropriate food sources, consumed in suitable proportions. The alkaline diet menu plays a vital role in achieving the desired outcomes of the diet. This article aims to elucidate the advantages of alkaline diets on our overall well-being, provide practical guidelines for effectively adopting this dietary approach, and furnish a comprehensive list of foods to consider incorporating into your alkaline diet menu.

The Historical Account of Human Dietary Patterns

The dietary habits of ancient humans starkly contrast with our modern food consumption patterns. In ancient times, humans predominantly subsisted on uncooked, plant-derived sustenance, occasionally incorporating infrequent, limited amounts of animal proteins into their diets. In contemporary times, the dietary consumption of animal proteins has significantly increased within the average human diet. Additionally, there has been a significant increase in our consumption of heavily processed and artificial food products that contain an abundance of detrimental toxins detrimental to the overall well-being of our bodies. The overconsumption of salts, artificial sweeteners, and food additives contributes to the heightened acidity levels found in our contemporary diets. This heightened consumption of acid disrupts the body's innate equilibrium, which ideally rests at a healthy pH level of 7.3. Consequently, it impairs multiple crucial physiological functions within the body.

The Mechanisms Underlying the Functionality of Alkaline Diets

By deliberately regulating the equilibrium between acidity and alkalinity in your body, you can derive numerous advantages in terms of your overall well-being. The effects of heightened energy levels and shedding of excess weight will become readily apparent to individuals who have recently restored their body's equilibrium by reducing acidity. By adhering to a dietary regimen consisting of approximately 75% alkaline foods and limiting acidic foods to only 25%, one can restore the body to its optimal, innate condition. Furthermore, by utilizing alkaline water in the preparation of acidic foods, one can significantly mitigate their potential to cause acidification within the body. The implementation of an alkaline diet operates to alleviate the strain exerted on one's liver, kidneys, and other bodily organs resulting from an excessively acidic (toxic) internal environment.

Your Menu for the Alkaline Diet

Please find below a compilation of various food selections that we highly recommend for the adoption of an alkaline diet. Although it is necessary to include acidic foods in a balanced diet, it is important to restore their levels to those which our bodies initially adapted to.

Alkaline Fruits:

apples

bananas

blackberries

dates

oranges

pineapple

raisins

Alkaline Vegetables:

broccoli

cabbage

carrots

cauliflower

celery

eggplant

mushrooms

squash

turnips

It is recommended that the consumption of acidic foods should not exceed 25% of one's dietary intake. Herein lies an inventory of food categories characterized by their acidic nature. Please be mindful that each category presented below contains both highly acidic foods and those that lean towards the alkaline side.

Acidic Foods:

meat

cheese

legumes

grains

nuts

select fruits

select vegetables

A Compilation of Acidic, Alkaline, and Neutral Food Items

A well-balanced nutritional regimen is a fundamental aspect contributing to optimal health. One method to guarantee a well-rounded diet is by consuming foods from each of the food groups, while another approach involves maintaining a balance between the consumption of acidic or acid-forming foods and alkaline foods. This facilitates the maintenance of your body's pH balance, a crucial aspect for ensuring optimal physiological functioning and mitigating the risk of diseases. Having knowledge of the food items that tend to create acidity, promote alkalinity, or have a neutral effect can aid in organizing your meals.

Acid-Forming Foods

Food items that contribute to an acidic internal environment encompass a wide range of items, such as processed foods, meat and fish products, rice, grains, sweeteners, breads, pastas, dairy products including cheese, caffeinated beverages, alcoholic beverages, and condiments. Certain nuts and seeds exhibit an acid-forming characteristic. Illustrative instances encompass beef, potato chips, salmon, chicken, and pork. Artificial sweeteners, as well as cane and beet sugars, barley syrup, processed honey, maple syrup, and molasses, all possess an acidic nature. Certain fruits and vegetables possess acid-forming properties, which encompass a variety of beans, dried-sulfured fruits, as well as blueberries and cranberries. The classification of acid-containing nuts encompasses a variety of selections such as walnuts, pecans, cashews, pistachios, macadamias, filberts, Brazil nuts, and peanuts. In addition, it should be noted that sunflower and pumpkin seeds have an acidic effect on the body. Mustard, ketchup, mayonnaise, and vinegar can be regarded as condiments with acidifying properties. Carbonated beverages, coffee, sweetened teas, fruit juices, beer, and wine can be characterized as acidic beverages.

Alkalizing Foods

Consuming an ample amount of alkaline-rich foods aids in the restoration of equilibrium in the body, counteracting the impact of acidic food items. The majority of fresh fruits and vegetables possess alkalizing properties. This encompasses lettuces, various varieties of potatoes, cruciferous vegetables encompassing broccoli, kale, Brussels sprouts, and cauliflower, herbs like parsley and dill, as well as carrots, beets, eggplant, and sprouts. In addition, sprouted beans possess alkalizing properties. Alkaline fruits encompass a variety of options such as avocados, pears, peaches, cherries, apples, various types of melons, bananas, dates, papayas, figs, and grapes. Certain dairy products possess alkaline properties, including buttermilk, raw milk, plain yogurt, and acidophilus milk. Amaranth and quinoa are grains with alkalizing properties, while almonds, chestnuts, and fresh coconut are nuts that have alkalizing effects. Additional alkaline foods that can be incorporated into one's diet are honey, kelp, tea, and egg yolks.

Neutral Foods

Neutral foods do not exhibit either acidic or alkaline properties upon consumption, thereby exerting a balanced impact on the body. Neutral food options consist of unseasoned, freshly churned butter; raw and unprocessed cream; unpasteurized cow's milk and whey; as well as margarine and various types of oils.

Establishing an Optimal Equilibrium

Merely because a food has acid-forming properties does not imply that it should be excluded from your diet. Incorporating acid-forming foods into your diet is crucial as they serve as valuable sources of essential nutrients like heart-healthy fatty acids derived from fish, and grains, which are rich in B vitamins. The crucial strategy lies in abstaining from consuming detrimental acid-forming foods such as potato chips, processed grains, sweeteners, and carbonated beverages, and instead opting for nourishing alternatives like lean meats, whole grains, and unflavored dairy products. It is highly recommended to consume ample amounts of alkaline fruits and vegetables. By adhering to the guidance provided by the U.S. Department of Agriculture, which advices allocating fifty percent of your plate to fruits and vegetables during every meal, you are taking significant strides towards improving your overall well-being.

Porridge Made With Quinoa, Served With Succulent Plums

Ingredients:

1 tbsp chia seeds
3-4 plums, sliced
½ tsp pink Himalayan salt
½ cup quinoa
1 ½ cups water
¼ tsp ground cinnamon

Preparation:

Transfer the quinoa into a saucepan of moderate size. Incorporate water and bring it to a state of boiling. Thoroughly mix the ingredients and then lower the heat to a moderate level. Cook for 3-4 minutes. Eliminate from the heat source and incorporate cinnamon, salt, and chia seeds through stirring.

Allow to cool thoroughly and carefully transfer to a suitable vessel for serving. Garnish with plums and present to your guests.

What Are Acidic Foods?

Hence, the acid-forming foods serve as the corollary to their alkaline counterparts. In any event, there is variability in the levels of acidity among these food items. This document exclusively delineates the acidic impact on the human body.

Examples of foods that are acid-forming include meat and sweet pastries. They exhibit no discernible sourness, but rather possess a savoury or sweet flavour. For instance, certain alkaline food items possess a sour flavor profile, like lemons.

When the body metabolizes acidic foods, it generates acidic byproducts. In addition, acidic foods exhibit a total of eight distinct characteristics.

To start with, foods that promote acid formation contain an abundance of acidic minerals. These minerals encompass phosphorus, sulphur, and chlorine, to provide several examples.

Furthermore, these foods contain a plentiful amount of amino acids that have the capacity to generate acid, specifically methionine and cysteine. The consumption of a substantial quantity of these amino acids leads to the production of sulphuric acid within the human body.

Additionally, it should be noted that foods that promote acidity do not have the inherent ability to trigger the production of alkaline substances within the body. They do not contain any acrid substances or substances that induce alkaline formation in the body.

Furthermore, it should be noted that acidic foods consist of numerous components that give rise to a substantial quantity of waste byproducts and residual substances during the process of metabolism. The aforementioned components encompass sugar, alcohol, and caffeine.

Additionally, acidic foods impede the process of acid breakdown in the body due to their inadequate content of essential vitamins, antioxidants, and other compounds that facilitate the breakdown process.

Additionally, alkaline foods differ in their water content as they contain minimal amounts. The consumption of alkaline foods, such as, can effectively serve as a remedy in cases of inadequate fluid intake. On the contrary, this is not the case with acidic foods. Consequently, the acids can be excreted with even less efficiency through the renal system.

In addition, it should be noted that the consumption of acidic foods can elicit a pro-inflammatory response due to their high saturation of fatty acids and comparatively low content of beneficial unsaturated and polyunsaturated fatty acids.

Moreover, these foods exert a detrimental impact on the gastrointestinal microbiota.

Consequently, the excretion of the remaining acids is further limited. Furthermore, compromised intestinal health gives rise to the development of bacterial elements which contribute to the occurrence of hyperacidity (toxins).

For the purpose of adhering to an alkaline diet, it is advisable to primarily consume alkaline foods. Hence, it is advisable to refrain from consuming foods that promote acid formation in order to establish a harmonious equilibrium between acidic and basic components.

Subsequently, there will be presented a compilation of specific instances of both alkaline and acidic foods.

Alkaline foods:

A variety of fruits, including apples, dragon fruit, pears, peaches, melons, mandarins, figs, dates, and oranges, both fresh and dried, can be found in the selection.

A diverse range of vegetables encompasses cauliflower, pumpkin, spinach, sweet potato, potato, carrots, celery, peppers, fresh peas, asparagus, and numerous other varieties.

Some of the herbs that may be included are dill, oregano, chives, coriander, thyme, cloves, rosemary, amongst others.

Examples of mushrooms include porcini, mushrooms, and chanterelles.

Germinated plants such as broccoli sprouts, radish sprouts, or fenugreek sprouts

Alkaline drinks:

Water

Unsweetened botanical or fruity infusion.

Water infused with a splash of freshly squeezed lemon juice or a small amount of apple cider vinegar

Vegetable juices pressed just before consumption

Fruit-based beverages or blended drinks containing greens.

Acid-forming foods:

Milk

Quark

Yoghurt

Wholemeal products

Cheese

Eggs

Meat and sausage

Fish and seafood

White flour products

Sugary drinks

Alcohol

Rice

Side Effects/Cautions

Before embarking on the alkaline diet, it is crucial to acquaint oneself with the accompanying adverse effects that may arise.

Now, let us delve into the specifics of each of them.

Deficiency

The dietary regimen excludes the intake of specific food categories that may result in nutritional inadequacies. This encompasses dairy products that facilitate calcium intake, as well as meat products that serve as a source of proteins for the body. It may be necessary to ingest nutritional supplements in order to counterbalance these deficiencies. You may consult your physician to determine whether or not it is necessary for you to take the supplements. Additionally, you have the option to choose natural alternatives derived from plants.

Expectant mothers" or "Pregnant women

It is imperative that pregnant women seek guidance from their healthcare professionals prior to embarking on the alkaline diet. As you may already be aware, the diet omits certain essential nutrients that may hold significance for your overall bodily well-being. The physician may offer more proficient guidance and inform you of supplementary dietary amendments required. If you previously adhered to the diet prior to your pregnancy, it will remain crucial for you to seek professional advice.

Allergies

Non-vegetarians who desire to adopt the dietary regimen must ensure the omission of any allergenic foods from their meals. If one possesses knowledge of their allergens, it enables them to abstain from their consumption. If you lack knowledge on the matter, you could begin by ingesting minimal portions as a means of ascertaining which substances are deemed safe for consumption.

Expectations

It is imperative to maintain realistic expectations regarding one's dietary regimen. You must allocate sufficient time for it to exert its desired effects on your physique. Anticipating immediate outcomes will only lead to disillusionment. If you commence the dietary regimen today, you should anticipate observing outcomes within a span of one month. Individuals who are afflicted with obesity may experience an extended period to achieve weight loss. However, you will promptly notice the onset of several essential transformations in your physique, such as the development of radiant skin, resilient nails, and lustrous hair.

Pomegranate Smoothie

Ingredients

1/2 cup pomegranate arils
2 grapefruits, peeled and deseeded
1 cup coconut water
3 large collard leaves, stems removed

Directions

Incorporate grapefruits, pomegranate, collard leaves, and coconut water into a blender and blend until a smooth consistency is achieved.

Serve and enjoy. Incorporate a small amount of Stevia, should you desire.

Enhanced Energy Levels

Ensuring proper cellular functioning is imperative for an individual's overall vitality. In the event that the phones are not efficacious, they exhibit diminished efficacy in facilitating the absorption and transport of oxygen within the organism.

This can lead to overall fatigue and a lack of energy. The pH level of the body can also impact a cell's ability to generate adenosine triphosphate (ATP), a crucial component for the body's energy level. This process typically occurs within the intracellular organelle known as the mitochondria. Should the pH level of the body become overly acidic, the effectiveness of this procedure is compromised.

Enhanced dental health and periodontal well-being

When the pH level of the body exceeds an acidic threshold, it follows that the acidity in the mouth will also be significantly elevated. Regrettably, in instances where the oral acidity level surpasses the norm, it can facilitate accelerated microorganism growth. Microorganisms have the potential to give rise to a multitude of concerns within the oral cavity, such as periodontal disease and halitosis.

An atypical condition characterized by the presence of corrosive substances and microorganisms within the oral cavity will also heighten an individual's susceptibility to dental cavity development. Many individuals observe a shift in their overall oral health upon transitioning to a diet regimen that promotes an alkaline pH level within the body.

Enhanced Immune Function

When cells are in a healthy state, they are adequately capable of assimilating the necessary nutrients. Solid cells also demonstrate significant efficacy in the elimination of waste materials.

If cellular functionality becomes compromised in any manner, their efficacy in carrying out such functions significantly diminishes. Consequently, inescapable organisms possess a greater likelihood of exerting an impact on these cells.

When the pH balance of the body becomes excessively acidic, cellular functionality is compromised and unable to reach its optimal level. The aforementioned circumstances may lead to males experiencing illnesses, infections, or even developing tumors, particularly when their diet is predominantly acidic in comparison to alkaline.

Diminished Pain and Inflammation

Magnesium is among the minerals employed by the human body to regulate excessive acidity. If one consumes a diet that induces an acidic effect, the body is compelled to utilize a greater amount of magnesium in order to neutralize it.

Nevertheless, magnesium also plays a significant role as a beneficial supplement in supporting the functionality of joints and tissues within the human body. By adhering to a dietary regimen that exerts an alkaline influence on the body rather than an acidic influence, an increased amount of magnesium will be made available to alleviate joint pain and inflammation.

Slower Aging

When cells are exposed to an acidic environment, their efficiency diminishes significantly. This attenuation of efficacy can impair a cell's ability to undergo self-repair, thereby resulting in premature aging.

Premature aging can also occur when cells are deprived of adequate oxygen and are unable to effectively eliminate toxins. Following a fundamental dietary regimen can contribute to the prevention of such circumstances.

Enhanced cellular functionality leads to a rejuvenated physical appearance. Additionally, as an added benefit, a water-soluble dietary program will also aid in maintaining optimal weight.

The Impact Of An Alkaline Diet On Weight Management

The underlying principle of the alkaline diet is based on the concept that as the pH level of our body is moderately alkaline, typically ranging from 7.36 to 7.44, our dietary choices should align with this by favoring a slightly alkaline composition. A diet that lacks equilibrium due to excessive consumption of acid-forming foods such as animal protein, caffeine, sugar, and processed foods typically disrupts this equilibrium. It has the potential to diminish the body's alkaline mineral reserves, namely sodium, potassium, magnesium, and calcium, rendering individuals susceptible to chronic and degenerative ailments.

The regulation of our internal chemical equilibrium primarily depends on the functioning of our lungs, kidneys, intestines, and skin. In order for essential physiological processes to take place, it is imperative that our body maintains an appropriate pH level. The parameter that denotes the level of acidity or alkalinity of a substance is referred to as pH. Sufficient alkaline reserves are necessary for optimal pH adjustment. The human body requires oxygen, water, and minerals with acid-buffering properties in order to efficiently maintain optimal pH levels and swiftly eliminate waste products.

The excessive acidification of the body is the fundamental factor behind all illnesses. Soda is likely the most acidic consumable, with a pH level of 2.5. It surpasses the acidity of neutral water by a factor of 50,000, requiring the consumption of 32 glasses of neutral water to neutralize the acidity of a single glass of soda.

A diet rich in alkaline foods and consumption of alkaline water are essential for ensuring the body receives the necessary nutrients to counteract acids and toxins present in the blood, lymph, and tissues. Moreover, this practice serves to fortify both the immune and organ systems.

The majority of vegetables and fruits possess a greater abundance of alkaline-forming elements compared to other types of food. The extent to which an individual incorporates a higher proportion of green foods into their diet directly corresponds to the magnitude of the health benefits they can attain. These plant-based foods possess purifying and alkalizing properties that benefit the body, whereas refined and processed foods have the potential to elevate unhealthy acidity levels and toxin accumulation.

However, it is important to note that an excessive amount of alkaline can also be detrimental to your well-being. It is imperative to possess the requisite understanding of maintaining a harmonious equilibrium between alkaline and acidic foods within one's dietary consumption. Upon consumption, the alkaline food and water undergo almost instantaneous neutralization by the hydrochloric acid present in the stomach. The maintenance of a harmonious equilibrium between alkaline and acidic foods is imperative for optimal functioning of your organs.

In terms of pH levels, a nutritious and well-rounded diet tends to be more alkaline than acidic. In accordance with your blood type, the dietary composition should consist of 60 to 80% alkaline foods and 20 to 40% acidic foods. Typically, the A and AB blood types necessitate the adoption of an alkaline diet, whereas the O and B blood types necessitate a higher consumption of animal products in their dietary intake. It is important to consider that if one is experiencing pain, they may be acidic.

The process of adopting an alkaline diet necessitates a change in one's perspective on food. It is advantageous to experiment with novel flavors and textures while making incremental modifications and enhancing established practices.

The diet adhering to alkaline principles and its correlation with weight reduction.
In order to determine the potential efficacy of adopting an Alkaline Diet for weight loss, it is imperative to gain a comprehensive understanding of the mechanisms by which the diet operates, as well as the intricate interplay between various food groups within this dietary framework.

In the first place, it is imperative to comprehend that every single food item consumed undergoes complete metabolism within our bodies, resulting in the formation of an ash residue. This residual ash can exhibit neutral, acidic, or alkaline properties.

Moreover, it is crucial to comprehend that the cells in a well-functioning organism are immersed in an alkaline solution. Acidosis, or excessive acidification of bodily fluids and tissues, results in a disruption of cellular equilibrium, potentially leading to illness and disease, as well as the accumulation of excess fat in the body tissues.

Chapter Five: Maximizing the Effectiveness of the Alkaline Diet

One will observe that the alkaline diet presents a minimal learning curve. The emphasis lies in modifying one's dietary routines rather than adopting a novel eating plan. As per the analysis of professionals, it requires a period of 21 days to alleviate a habit. Hence, one should anticipate a span of several weeks to adapt and become accustomed to the new dietary regimen. It is possible to encounter certain mild side effects during the days and weeks following the elimination of sugar, caffeine, and other nutritionally disadvantageous foods. The adverse effects typically subside within a few days. Numerous individuals have discovered that the consumption of a small amount of lemon-infused water is effective in mitigating the majority of the associated symptoms.

The subsequent observations are a selection of phenomena that you might potentially discern within the initial 72-hour timeframe subsequent to commencing your diet regimen and abstaining from deleterious food items.

Headache

Irritability

Nausea

Tiredness

Anxiousness

You may encounter moments of notable enticement, which may occasionally lead to succumbing to the consumption of a candy bar or a similar food item that does not strictly adhere to the principles of the alkaline diet. That is okay. It will not significantly compromise your health. It is important to restrict the consumption of those small indulgences. By abstaining from indulgence, one merely intensifies their desire for it. In the forthcoming chapter, you will discover a selection of recipes designed to appease your indulgent desires without compromising your dietary goals. Make an effort to seek out nutritious alternatives for the item you desire.

Recommended Food Sources for an Alkaline-Enriched Dietary Regimen

Below, you will find a comprehensive compilation of food items that are highly recommended and regarded as suitable for consumption while adhering to the alkaline diet. Foods that elicit an alkaline response consist of uncooked fruits and vegetables, seeds, nuts, herbal infusions, and botanicals. Attempt to replace the items you typically consume with alternatives from the provided list.

Almond milk

Broccoli

Cauliflower

Tofu

Chestnuts

Apples

Bananas

Melons

Berries

Cucumbers

Cold pressed olive oil

Sweet potatoes

Lentils

Wild rice

These food items are recommended for inclusion in your dietary regimen. Undoubtedly, the consumption of fresh fruits and vegetables is highly beneficial for one's well-being. If fresh produce is not readily available, choosing frozen alternatives over canned options is recommended in order to avoid the inclusion of syrups typically used during the canning process. As evident to your observation, the mention of meat is conspicuously absent. Nevertheless, poultry can be considered periodically. A plant-based dietary regimen is indeed commendable and currently enjoys significant popularity in contemporary times. You will find an abundance of meat alternatives available in your local grocery store, as well as in the majority of dining establishments.

Foods that should be minimized due to their potential for acid production encompass grains, fast food, processed food, dairy products, the majority of meat, legumes, and fish. In addition, it is imperative to abstain from consuming alcohol, despite certain recommendations that may endorse the occasional consumption of a draft beer. Sugars exhibit high levels of acidity and are recommended to be abstained from.

Tips to Being Successful

Numerous individuals have preceded you in pursuing this dietary regimen and have achieved notable success in doing so. One can acquire a wealth of knowledge from individuals who have experienced the trials and tribulations of learning through difficult circumstances, which enlighten us about effective and ineffective approaches. Please peruse these recommendations which can assist you in adhering to your alkaline diet.

Prepare your meals in advance. This will facilitate a reduction in your inclination or necessity to opt for expeditious and probably detrimental alternatives. Prepare your weekly meals ahead of time on a designated day of rest and store them in the freezer. This method offers a significant time-saving opportunity through the practice of preparing meals in larger quantities.

When dining at a buffet establishment, one should promptly proceed towards the salad bar and partake in an ample portion of verdant greens and an abundant variety of vegetables. You will have a decreased inclination to approach the hot display case, where the foods known to cause acid reflux are typically found.

Consume herbal tea as a replacement for coffee during the morning hours. Coffee is strictly prohibited when adhering to the alkaline diet.

Ensure that you have readily available access to carbonated water in times of craving for a sugary beverage. For added flavoring, consider incorporating a small amount of lemon juice or a dash of stevia.

When placing an order for a salad at a dining establishment, kindly request the dressing to be served separately.

Replace cow's milk with alternatives such as soy or almond milk.

Replace mashed or baked potatoes with wild rice

When you experience the inclination for snacking, engage in physical activity. Engage in a brief stroll encompassing the vicinity, ascend a set of stairs, or perform a series of yoga postures within your workplace to effectively combat the desire.

Ensure that you obtain an ample amount of sleep each night to counteract the midday decline in energy that prompts you to opt for beverages and snacks laden with sugar.

When preparing meals, substitute olive oil for butter or other types of oil.

Incorporate salads into your dietary regimen – It is worth noting that salads offer significant nutritional value for various reasons, including their ability to promote an alkaline balance within the body. Optimal ingredients for usage would encompass dark-hued salad greens, such as uncooked spinach, of significant nutritional value. Additionally, iceberg lettuce can also be utilized. It is advisable to incorporate nourishing fats in your salad as well. This can be achieved by integrating one to two slices of avocado. Drizzle the salad with a dressing made primarily from olive oil. This will enable you to savor a delectable meal that has the dual benefit of promoting an alkaline pH in your body and facilitating the maintenance of a desirable weight.

Exercise caution in the cooking process to prevent excessive cooking of vegetables, as prolonged cooking can result in a loss of their nutritional value. If feasible, consume the majority of your vegetables in their uncooked state. An alternative method would be to steam them gently as well. This proves advantageous in the case of desiring to uphold their alkaline nature.

Refrain from consuming processed grains and sugar as they can significantly contribute to the acidification of your body. Initiate the reduction of your consumption of noodles, industrially processed cereals, baked goods, and bread. Direct your attention towards incorporating unprocessed grains such as millet, amaranth, quinoa, and wild rice into your diet.

Reduce your consumption of dairy products and meat as they also contribute to the acidification of the body. One may opt for alternative protein sources such as soy cheese, soymilk, soybeans, almonds, goat cheese, and goat milk as substitutes for acid-forming foods.

Incorporate fruits into your dietary regimen - The efficacy of an alkaline diet may fail to meet desired expectations without the inclusion of fruits. Direct your attention towards incorporating papaya, watermelon, citrus fruits, blueberries, apples, and mangoes into your dietary regimen. You are also permitted to consume raisins. Exercise caution when incorporating fruits into your dietary routine, as certain fruits may exhibit acidifying properties. Among the fruits that should be avoided due to their acidifying properties are blackberries, cranberries, and prunes.

Avoid the use of artificial sweeteners, as they have the potential to detrimentally affect the pH balance of your body. The most optimal and healthful alternatives to artificial sweeteners consist of natural Stevia, unprocessed maple sugar, and unrefined sugar. These products are highly suitable for individuals adhering to an alkaline diet. Additionally, it is recommended to substitute conventional soft drinks, both diet and regular, with herbal or green tea as this substitution can effectively enhance the equilibrium of your pH level.

Acquire the ability to harmonize and balance food combinations - Electing to adhere to an alkaline diet should not necessitate forsaking all preferred acid-forming foods. It should be observed that moderation is of utmost importance in this dietary regimen. It is imperative that you maintain moderation in the consumption of acidifying foods. One may also combine alkaline and acidic foods in order to promote optimal nutrition and digestion. One may utilize a food combination chart as it can assist in the proper pairing and blending of foods.

Maintain proper hydration – Adequate fluid intake is imperative in adhering to an alkaline diet. It is advisable to consume approximately six to eighteen cups of water on a daily basis. In addition, one may rehydrate by consuming lemon-infused water. To prepare it, simply incorporate freshly extracted lemon juice into two cups of strained, tepid water. This remedy effectively facilitates the purification of your digestive system, accelerates your metabolism, and regulates the surplus acidity. Although it is indeed a fact that lemons possess acidic properties in their inherent state, the mixture of water and lemon remains predisposed to alkalinity upon ingestion. Organic herbal infusions such as nettle, peppermint, and Rooibos possess the capacity to effectively replenish your body's hydration levels.

Strive for a gradual and efficient transition – There is no need to exert pressure upon oneself to adhere strictly to the alkaline diet, particularly if one has not yet embraced it wholeheartedly. If you exert undue pressure on yourself, there is a significant probability of experiencing failure within a mere span of one week. Take everything slowly. One advantage of adhering to the alkaline diet is its lack of restrictiveness and difficulty. Indeed, it is straightforward. Simply refrain from attempting to achieve perfection from the initial stages. Adopting a gradual approach can facilitate the acclimation of your body to your new lifestyle, thereby simplifying the process of learning, experimenting, and discovering suitable meals. Additionally, there is an increased likelihood of adhering to the dietary regimen over an extended period of time.

Engage in respiratory exercises - You can anticipate enhanced effectiveness of the alkaline diet by complementing it with uncomplicated breathing techniques. Engage in these exercises on a daily basis, preferably completing them once or twice. These exercises have the potential to facilitate the elimination of acidic substances from your body. This practice also serves to alkalize your system, as it allows you to pause, unwind, engage in visualization, and concentrate your thoughts.

Manage stress levels – It is crucial to recognize that the impact of your emotions on acidity is significantly stronger compared to the acidic content of the beverages and meals you consume. An excessive amount of stress can induce various unfavorable physiological responses within the body. It is highly probable that you will experience discomfort and soreness in various areas of your physique. Make an effort to alleviate stress periodically to facilitate the effectiveness of the alkaline diet in enhancing your overall well-being.

Indulge in occasional rewards – It is important to periodically acknowledge and indulge in pleasurable moments to avoid the perception of self-deprivation in your conscious mind. This can assist in fostering the notion that you retain the permission to consume specific foods, consequently mitigating your cravings. Be certain to consistently uphold willpower and exercise discipline at all times. You must refrain from indulging in excessive self-indulgence. It would be prudent to select your most preferred indulgences and allow yourself an opportunity to savor them, albeit in moderation.

By implementing the suggestions outlined in this chapter, you will discover enhanced facilitation in adhering to the alkaline diet.

Acid To Alkaline Diet

What precisely is an acid alkaline diet?

Many individuals have been encountering challenges in discovering the most suitable dietary regimen for their needs. One of the prevailing misconceptions that these individuals possess is their aspiration for weight reduction. They neglect to place adequate emphasis on the importance of maintaining good health. If you wish to ascertain the optimal dietary regimen that is tailored to your specific needs, it is advisable to ensure its nutritional value and refrain from engaging in practices that may have detrimental effects on your physiological well-being.

The concept of maintaining a pH-balanced diet is gaining increasing attention in contemporary discourse; nevertheless, a large portion of the population remains uninformed about its nature and implications. Individuals who pass away prematurely, experience health issues, or struggle with obesity, typically exhibit a highly acidic internal environment. Conversely, individuals who live to advanced ages without significant health problems possess an internal environment that is characterized by a more alkaline nature.

In contemporary Western society, a significant majority of individuals lead an exceedingly unhealthy way of life, primarily characterized by the consumption of unhealthy and nutrient-poor food, as well as consistent exposure to various factors that significantly detrimentally affect our well-being. This lifestyle stands in stark opposition to the principles of the alkaline diet. In accordance with the findings of the World Health Organization (WHO), the global population of obese adults exceeds one billion individuals, approximately three hundred million of whom are classified as clinically obese. This statistic is concerning and is experiencing a significant increase on a daily basis.

As a healthcare practitioner, I am frequently approached by individuals seeking advice on the most effective methods for maintaining good health. I frequently inform my patients that in order to maintain a state of good health, prevent excessive weight gain, mitigate the risk of severe diseases and ailments, and ultimately enjoy a long and vibrant life, it is imperative that we prioritize the monitoring and maintenance of an appropriate acid-alkaline balance in our diet.

By monitoring one's body's pH levels and adjusting one's diet accordingly to achieve a state of higher alkalinity than acidity, individuals may experience various benefits such as rapid weight loss through an accelerated fat disposal process, an increased lifespan, reduced stress levels, enhanced immune system function, improved quality of sleep, heightened energy levels, and a potential boost in libido.

These advantages in and of themselves are undoubtedly significant in terms of promoting good health, extending life expectancy, and cultivating overall happiness. By enabling the body to undergo detoxification through the adoption of an acid to alkaline diet, individuals also enhance their capacity to assimilate essential vitamins and minerals, thereby mitigating the risk of various detrimental ailments such as cancer and arthritis. With an increased level of alkalinity in the body, the alleviation of stress and pressure on the internal organs occurs, promoting the rejuvenation of the skin, bones, and cells, thereby contributing to a more youthful appearance.

Conversely, if an individual's body exhibits excessive acidity, they may readily encounter weight gain and retention of fat, accelerate the aging process, commonly experience fatigue, become more prone to various diseases and viruses, and foster an internal environment conducive to the proliferation of yeast and bacteria.

The majority of individuals residing in the Western world generally do not adhere to an acid to an alkaline diet and typically lean towards the acidic side.

This is primarily attributable to our dietary habits. Consuming items such as unhealthy snacks, hamburgers, carbonated beverages, indulging in excessive sugar, fried cuisine, artificially flavored fruit juices, imitation products, energy drinks, and processed foods are all factors that contribute to the acidity of our internal bodily environment.

There are also certain healthy food items that require caution, such as strawberries, mangoes, and peaches, due to their considerable sugar content, which consequently induces acidity within the body. Several additional unexpected contributors to the accumulation of acidity consist of rice, tuna, oats, and cheese. Therefore, it is advisable to restrict consumption of these food items while adhering to the alkaline diet.

This is one rationale behind the cruciality of understanding precisely which foods elicit an acid response versus those that promote alkalinity. Additional factors that contribute to the increased acidity of our bodies are various chemicals, tobacco, radiation, pesticides, artificial sweeteners, air pollution, alcohol, drugs, and stress.

The pH level of 7.4 is the optimal point to derive all the advantageous effects of alkalinity. In the event that there is a deviation of 3-4 units in your body, it will result in fatality. The pH scale can be delineated as such:

The value of zero represents the complete absence of acid/battery acid, specifically hydrochloric acid.

1 corresponds to gastric juices

The number two is equivalent to vinegar.

Three equals beer.

Four is equivalent to wine or tomato juice.

The numerical value of 5 represents the occurrence of precipitation in the form of rain.

The value of 6 is equal to that of milk.

Seven represents pure water.

The numerical value of 8 is equivalent to that of seawater.

Nine is equivalent to baking soda.

The numerical expression 10 can be represented as the combination of detergent and milk of magnesia.

Ammonia can be represented as 11, while lime water is another term used.

The numerical representation of "12" is equivalent to the chemical substance known as bleach.

The equation "13 equals lye" can be expressed in a more formal manner as "The numerical expression 13 is equivalent to the alphanumeric sequence lye."

The sum of 14 corresponds to the overall amount of Alkaline/Sodium Hydroxide.

The acid incorporated into the alkaline diet promotes maintenance of the body's pH level within the optimal range, approximately 7.4. The physiological response to maintaining this acid-alkaline equilibrium is both intriguing and captivating. When the acidity levels within your body become excessive, it initiates various processes aimed at achieving a more alkaline state.

When such a circumstance arises, the human body will retain a certain amount of acidic elements within its adipose tissue as a precautionary measure, effectively safeguarding the body against potential harm. Although this process is advantageous, it subsequently results in the body's retention of excess fat as a protective mechanism, thereby causing weight gain in individuals.

In instances of internal acidosis, the human body seeks alkaline sources outside of the bones and teeth, resulting in the fragility and deterioration of these skeletal structures. This can result in a variety of skeletal and dental disorders, such as arthritis and dental caries. This scenario would not occur if an individual were adhering to an acid-to-alkaline diet.

The accumulation of acid typically tends to migrate towards the least robust organs in your body, which are already susceptible to ailments, instead of dissipating towards your healthier organs. It resembles a group of wolves scouring the herd for the most vulnerable members, selectively targeting the easy prey.

When your less resilient organs become susceptible, it significantly facilitates the onset of grave illnesses, such as cancer. It is crucial to recognize that cancer cells enter a dormant state when the body's pH levels reach 7.4, which is the optimal pH level. This reiterates the significance of maintaining a healthy pH level within our bodies by adhering to the acid to alkaline diet.

In the presence of acidity within the system, it likewise impairs the purity of your bloodstream. Consequently, this hinders the blood type's capacity to efficiently transport oxygen to the tissues. Red blood cells are enshrouded by an unfavorable charge, which enables them to experience repulsive forces and navigate in the bloodstream with exceptional swiftness to accomplish their optimal functionality. However, when the acidity level is excessively high, the charged particles lose their negative charge and adhere to one another, resulting in significantly reduced movement.

Section 5: The Biological Catalysts for Digestion

Carbohydrates and lipids undergo initial digestion within the oral cavity, wherein they combine with salivary amylase and other digestive enzymes. Contrarily, proteins undergo digestion within the gastric environment.

Mouth

Amylase is secreted within the salivary glands and undergoes blending with food during mastication, facilitated by the movement of the tongue.

Stomach

The stomach assumes a crucial role in the process of food digestion by means of combining, grinding, or triturating the ingested food and amalgamating it with digestive enzymes that facilitate its breakdown. The stomach secretes gastric enzymes. Enzymes engage in a synergistic interaction with hormones and other compounds during the process of digestion.

These include:

Pepsin, responsible for the breakdown of proteins into peptides and amino acids,

Hydrochloric acid manufactured within the parietal cells exerts a bactericidal and virucidal effect on microorganisms present in the consumed food.

The mucous cells secrete mucin, which acts as a barrier to safeguard the stomach lining against the corrosive effect of gastric acids.

The hormone gastrin, which is secreted by the G cells located in the stomach, stimulates the secretion of hydrochloric acid as well as the intrinsic factor.

The Intrinsic Factor, synthesized within the gastric glands by the parietal cells, facilitates the binding of Vitamin B12, thereby safeguarding it against degradation caused by hydrochloric acid, in order to enable its optimal absorption.

assimilated within the ileum

Gastric lipase, along with lingual lipase, constitutes the primary acidic enzymes involved in the process of digestion. The pH of gastric lipase ranges from 3 to 6.

Pancreas

Pancreatic juice is synthesized within the pancreas and is subsequently transported to the small intestine via the pancreatic duct. After progressing into the small intestine, the digestion process persists until the food proceeds to the large intestines. Acidity causes pancreatitis.

Bile is produced by the liver and subsequently stored within the gall bladder. It traverses the bile duct in order to facilitate the breakdown of fats and proteins. The development of gallstones can be attributed to the acidic nature of bile, which elicits considerable discomfort.

Small intestine

Below are the digestive enzymes and hormones that are synthesized in the duodenum: "

Lactase

Sucrase

Maltase

Erepsin

Secretin

Gastric inhibitory peptide

Motilin

Cholecystokinin

Somatostatisin

Acidosis has an impact on the digestive enzymes, impairing their ability to carry out their physiological functions and subsequently disrupting the overall metabolism of the body. In order to optimize the efficacy of digestive enzymes and hormones, it is imperative to adopt an alkaline diet to decrease bodily fluids.

Chapter Five: An Examination of the pH Miracle
The pH Miracle represents an exemplary remedy that enhances bodily well-being, facilitates weight reduction, and effectively confronts

various ailments. Numerous individuals express dissatisfaction regarding their inability to think clearly, and the ph Miracle can effectively alleviate mental fogginess as well.

Could you please provide an explanation of the ph Miracle? It is simply a term used to describe a program devised by a medical professional aiming to restore your physical well-being. It is inherent to the functioning of our body to maintain an alkaline state continuously.

The ingestion of contemporary dietary substances, coupled with the incorporation of various additives into our food, results in an excessive accumulation of acidity within our bodily system. Excessive levels of acid in the body result in the disruptions of various bodily functions. When adhering to this program, the acid is effectively eliminated, allowing your body to return to its desired alkaline state.

This program is designed to facilitate weight loss and has demonstrated success in reversing conditions like diabetes and elevated cholesterol levels.

Visit your local health store and inquire about the innovative regimen capable of reinstating your body's optimal state of health, witness the transformative impact it can have on your well-being, and experience an overall enhancement in your quality of life.

Adopting this living and dietary program will augment the inclusion of vegetables in your daily intake, consequently providing your body with all the essential nutrients required for survival. Acquiring the knowledge and skills to restore the optimal alkaline level in your body will significantly transform your life.

The alkaline diet exhibits exceptional characteristics.

Numerous dietary regimens emphasize the identical food items that contribute to one's initial state of being overweight or ill. They kindly request individuals to reduce their consumption of those items, to increase their frequency of meals, or to combine them in alternative ways. Out of consideration for the creators of these diets, they are aware that a significant number of individuals are not inclined to make substantial modifications for the betterment of their well-being. We prefer a diet that primarily consists of processed and refined foods, including meat, sugar, and alcoholic beverages. The creators of the diet are merely striving to assist individuals in facilitating effortless modifications.

We have become accustomed to consuming food in this manner, and it is not solely our responsibility. The profit-driven food processing corporations have a vested interest in ensuring that we continue to consume in this manner. In this sector of the food industry, the level of profitability far surpasses that of the production of fundamental agricultural products such as fruits and vegetables.

Therefore, once more, I affirm that this diet is indeed distinct. If those alternative diets had proven effective, you would currently experience a state of being slender, robust, and full of vitality, thereby rendering this article unnecessary for your perusal. A dietary alteration would be unnecessary for you.

Presented herewith is an incomplete inventory of sustenance which one may freely consume within the framework of an alkaline diet:

Fresh fruits and freshly prepared juices

Fresh vegetables and fruit juices

Cooked veggies

Certain legumes and soybeans

Consume lean sources of protein, such as poultry and fish, along with a selection of eggs.

Certain grains

Nutrients derived from healthy fats and various types of nuts

It may come as a revelation to discover that certain vegetables and fruits are more beneficial for one's health than others.

"You are permitted to consume restricted amounts of these food and beverage items:

Dairy

Numerous prevalent cereal crops

Processed foods and refined sugars.

Substances of Alcohol and Caffeine

What is the experience of adhering to the alkaline diet, and what outcomes can one anticipate?

Similar to any modification in diet or lifestyle, one will experience a period of adaptation. However, due to the fact that you are consuming the cleanest fuel, which is highly desired by your body, unlike numerous dietary regimes, you will never experience hunger. Additionally, you have the opportunity to consume as much food as you desire until you have reached a point of contentment. In addition, calorie counting will not be necessary. And you will have the opportunity to indulge in a diverse assortment of options, ensuring that you never tire of the culinary experience.

Consider an alkaline diet as a form of "juice cleanse" for the body. However, it is not as drastic. You are consuming nutritionally rich and easily digestible foods that your body naturally desires. When the body is supplied with the essential nutrients it urgently requires, one's appetite ceases. And there is no cause for concern regarding unappealing vegetables, as there is an abundance of delectable recipes readily available online and in literature.

Given the myriad of dietary regimens available, what are the reasons to contemplate adopting an alternative approach such as the alkaline diet?

When adhered to correctly, one can anticipate a more effortless reduction of body fat compared to traditional methods. Numerous testimonials are available wherein individuals have reported a weight loss of more than two pounds per week. (And such a significant amount of weight would not be advisable in most dietary programs.) Additionally, your skin will regain its suppleness, your energy levels will elevate, and you will experience a rejuvenated sense of youthfulness.

Additionally, the alkaline diet accomplishes two significant objectives that conventional diets do not.

1. It offers enhanced nourishment to the cells of your body.

2. It possesses inherent properties that facilitate cellular detoxification and purification as well.

These two pieces of information are responsible for the efficacy and safety of an alkaline diet.

There is an abundance of unconventional dietary plans available in the market that make claims of facilitating weight loss. Regrettably, an examination of the nutritional composition of these dietary plans reveals a notorious deficiency. If weight loss is a goal, it is advisable to pursue it by adhering to a nourishing dietary regimen that promotes overall well-being, rather than solely focusing on achieving a thinner physique. The adoption of an alkaline diet represents a wholesome method for achieving weight loss, fostering sustained vitality, well-being, and motivation to shed excess weight.

Gaining a Profound Comprehension of the Alkaline Diet

An alkaline diet distinguishes itself from other dietary approaches by placing major emphasis on the impact of foods on the body's acidity or alkalinity. When food undergoes digestion and metabolic processes in the human body, it generates what is commonly known as an 'alkaline residue' or 'acidic residue.' The initial pH of the food does not contribute to the ultimate physiological impact in the body.

Indeed, certain food items with high acidity, such as citrus fruits, actually have an alkalizing effect when consumed. When an individual consumes a higher proportion of alkaline foods as opposed to acidic foods, it becomes possible to modulate the body's pH to an optimal level of approximately 7.3. While this degree of alkalinity may not be significantly elevated, it is adequate to yield numerous positive effects on one's well-being.

Implementing an Alkaline Diet for Weight Reduction

Numerous individuals endeavor to adopt trendy or quick-fix diets in pursuit of weight loss. These dietary regimens may yield initial outcomes, yet in the long run, this approach can prove to be an exceedingly detrimental method for achieving weight loss. Moreover, a considerable number of individuals tend to regain the weight once they discontinue their stringent dietary regimen.

The utilization of an acidic dietary regimen for the purpose of weight management and control necessitates a more extensive modification of one's lifestyle. The outcomes may not manifest immediately; nevertheless, there is a higher probability for the weight to remain stable and not be regained. An alkaline diet consists of abundant quantities of food that naturally possess low caloric content, such as the majority of vegetables and fruits. Numerous food items that possess elevated levels of fat and calories also have an acidifying effect. Consequently, the elimination of such foods from one's diet will lead to the occurrence of a natural and healthy reduction in weight. These food items encompass red meat, nutritionally dense foods high in fats, dairy products such as whole milk and cheese with elevated fat content, refined sugar, carbonated beverages, and alcoholic beverages.

After discontinuing the consumption of these foods, your physical well-being will significantly improve, as your body will experience greater health, reduced acidity levels, and noticeable weight loss throughout this period. Due to the diet's healthful nature, it can be adhered to for an extended duration. Indeed, numerous individuals who embark on an alkaline diet exclusively for the purpose of weight loss discover a plethora of other advantages. An enhanced level of physical energy, heightened immunity, and a comprehensive enhancement in health and well-being are among the numerous advantages one could attain through the adoption of an alkaline diet.

The Efficacy Of Alkaline Diets In Promoting Substantial Weight Loss

Presently, the global prevalence of obesity and overweight poses significant challenges. The prevalence of obesity exhibits a substantial correlation with the high consumption of fast food and processed food items. Contemporary dining commonly consists of processed carbohydrates, sugars, alcoholic beverages, as well as meat and dairy products. These food items elicit a highly acidic response in the body. Processed and fast foods have an acidic nature, resulting in acid formation within the body. The correlation exists between the rise in bodily acidity and the accumulation of adipose tissue, which serves to safeguard the crucial organs against heightened acid levels within the body.

"Individuals grappling with excessive weight may have

encountered or experimented with numerous weight reduction programs or products.' The one thing that most of these weight loss programs do not address is the cause of being overweight. The underlying issue of weight concerns will be effectively tackled through the implementation of alkaline diets, as elaborated upon in the subsequent section. An additional obstacle encountered by individuals who grapple with weight-related concerns pertains to maintaining persistent levels of optimum energy throughout the entirety of the day. Certain individuals resort to consuming snacks and beverages that are strongly acidic in nature, consequently resulting in weight gain.

Obesity and overweightness are correlated with a multitude of indicators of poor health, including but not limited to fatigue, diabetes, edema, cardiovascular issues, musculoskeletal discomfort, and an array of chronic conditions associated with one's lifestyle. Furthermore, it is disheartening for one to continuously endure the dissatisfaction of not attaining and appreciating the physique they aspire to, and which they truly merit. Another consequence of imbalanced body pH is the acceleration of aging, resulting in a premature appearance and signs of aging.

Alkaline diets possess the potential to bring about significant changes in both body composition and overall well-being. Alkaline diets have been embraced as a viable weight loss regimen, demonstrating substantial efficacy and long-term sustainability. Alkaline diets are inherently natural and highly secure in their application. We are regrettably not consuming an adequate quantity of alkaline-forming foods such as fresh produce, vegetables, nuts, and legumes.

The human body sustains a meticulous equilibrium with a pH

level of 7.36, exhibiting a mildly alkaline nature. An alteration in the body's pH level towards acidity induces a modification in the chemical composition of the body.

Nevertheless, the eradication of the acidic milieu within the body signifies that the adipose tissue amassed therein will be expunged in due course, as its purpose of serving as a repository for acidic residue is rendered superfluous. Alkaline diets effectively reduce food cravings due to the inherent ability of alkaline forming elements in foods to neutralize body acidity. After the alkaline diet has successfully alkalized the internal environment of the body, it prepares the body to eliminate the accumulated acid waste and effectively metabolize the stored fat. By adhering to alkaline diets, the body's pH level can also be harmonized towards a mildly alkaline state. As a result, each bodily organ operates more effectively, promoting a robust metabolism and enabling simplified management of weight.

When an optimal pH balance is attained through consumption of alkaline food and adoption of alkaline dietary practices, the body naturally settles at its ideal weight, cravings for food diminish, blood sugar levels return to a healthy range, and, finally, there is a significant and sustained improvement in energy levels. Moreover, individuals acquire knowledge regarding the manner in which specific food varieties contribute to the development of an acidic internal environment in the body. As a result, they develop an understanding and subsequently modify their dietary habits to effectively facilitate weight management.

Defining Your Objectives: Establishing your Purpose

Engaging in introspective reflection facilitates the establishment of objectives and elucidates the motives behind selecting a course, while numerous factors function as catalysts in the decision-making process that guides pathway selection. For parents, setting an exemplary example for their children is regarded as a matter of great importance. The restoration of well-being serves as the principal incentive for those who are unwell. For individuals who are obese, achieving a weight that is considered acceptable becomes the decisive criteria.

Regardless of the impetus, expressing it in written form serves to establish a focal point and a frame of reference in pursuit of the objective. Prior to commencing, allocate a brief span of time to document these factors in accordance with the SMART principle, as it facilitates the systematic breakdown of goals into more feasible and achievable segments. Engaging in writing facilitates adherence to the principles of simplicity, measurability, attainability, realism, and time specificity within the process.

Provided toward the conclusion of this publication is a meal plan spanning ten days, engineered to initiate the process and furnish substantiation of the efficacy of the alkaline diet. The ten-day strategy delineates a plan aligning with the SMART framework, illustrating that offering a constructive reaction to the prevailing conditions yields a gratifying result. This literary work, coupled with the comprehensive ten-day program, offers an abundance of diversity, rendering it intriguing and supplying adequate sustenance when meticulously accompanied.

When establishing objectives for weight reduction, it is crucial to place greater emphasis on the procedure rather than the end result. Outcome goals are established with a primary emphasis on the ultimate outcome. To clarify, the objective of shedding 10 pounds is centered on the end result. Although this objective is not inherently unfavourable, it fails to provide guidance on attaining said objective.

The establishment of objectives is a pivotal determinant in determining individual success and failure. The establishment of appropriate objectives will prove advantageous in numerous respects. Moreover, verifiable evidence demonstrates that individuals who establish concrete objectives are twice as likely to actualize their aspirations compared to those who attempt to do so without any specific goals in place. Consider it akin to a navigational guide. Should you embark on a journey, it is imperative to have a well-structured itinerary that serves as a navigational aid, facilitating your progression.

Adhering to the alkaline diet is a process that necessitates the establishment of goals, which will serve as a compass to steer you towards the ultimate achievement of success. Goals form the bedrock for effecting enduring transformations. They will determine whether you achieve success or face failure.

Chapter 5: The Pursuit of Scientific Inquiry

This chapter will present a comprehensive array of relevant research materials to substantiate the claims of the alkaline diet. The alkaline diet can be regarded as more than a passing trend conceptualized by a single nutritionist, as it demonstrates a limited degree of efficacy. This dietary regimen has undergone extensive scrutiny and evaluation across various scientific and research domains.

Investigation into the influence of dietary acid load on renal function, susceptibility to osteoporosis, and incidence of fractures among elderly males and females. Jia, L. Byberg, B. Lindholm, T. E. Larsson, L. Lind, K. Michaelsson, J. J. Carrero

This research focused on compromised renal function. It demonstrates a decrease in the capacity to eliminate excessive dietary acid. The researchers conducted an inquiry into the relationship connecting the dietary acid load and the bone mineral density, commonly referred to as BMD. It also encompasses the topic of osteoporosis and the associated risk of fractures.

"The effects of enhanced fruit and vegetable intake on the excretion of cortisol and cortisone in the 24-hour urine collection of children." - J.

Esche, L. Shi, A. Sanchez-Guijo, M.F. Hartmann, S. Wudy, T. Remer

Within the scope of this investigation, the alkalization process on various young adults was facilitated by the administration of mineral salt, resulting in a notable reduction in parameters associated with the excretion of glucocorticoid metabolites. The researchers examined the impacts of fruits and vegetables on the secretion of stress hormones throughout a duration of 24 hours.

"The impact of dietary acid load and milk-induced metabolic acidosis on human insulin resistance." - Rebecca S. The authors of this piece are Williams, Pinar Kozan, and Dorit Samocha-Bonet.

This research pertains to the Western dietary patterns and the elevated levels of dietary acidity.

142

This demonstrates that elevated levels of dietary acidity over a prolonged period can lead to a reduction in blood pH referred to as milk metabolic acidosis, among other consequences.

What are the advantages of adhering to the Alkaline Diet?

The widely followed Alkaline Diet, originating in the 20th century, is based on the premise that increased acidity in bodily fluids amplifies the vulnerability of the body to a range of ailments. Several examples of these conditions encompass urinary tract infections, kidney stones, as well as osteoporosis attributable to the acid-induced deterioration of bone strength in the body. By refraining from the consumption of foods with high acidity levels such as meats, cheese, and similar items, individuals can enhance their general well-being and reinstate the equilibrium between acid and alkaline levels in the body. By implementing these modifications, the Alkaline Diet presents dietary and lifestyle alterations that, albeit diverging from the norm familiar to the average American, offer a multitude of advantages.

One of the primary advantages of ensuring that your body maintains a state of equilibrium in terms of that balance is the reduced susceptibility to debilitating ailments. Some of the factors encompassed within this category are prolonged ailments, exhaustion, and the detrimental consequences linked to an increase in body mass. Once the pH levels in the blood have been effectively regulated, as is the intended outcome of adhering to the Alkaline Diet, essential minerals like calcium and magnesium are introduced into the bloodstream. This, in consequence, serves to enhance the integrity of bones and teeth, from which the body would extract minerals when acidity levels exceed optimal thresholds. The Alkaline Diet effectively fosters the general well-being and fortification of numerous vital elements within our physiological systems.

An additional advantageous aspect of the Alkaline Diet is its ability to effectively revitalize energy levels. Individuals with an excess of acidity in their physiological systems, leading to weight gain, may experience symptoms such as fatigue and diminished levels of energy. Enhancing the intake of alkaline-forming foods can effectively enhance our immune system, optimize our energy levels, and rejuvenate vitality, thereby enabling our bodies to combat diseases and illnesses more effectively. Furthermore, due to the fact that yeast flourishes in acidic environments, individuals adhering to the Alkaline Diet are consequently at reduced susceptibility to the occurrence of yeast infections.

Despite the limited number of medical tests and research validating the beneficial effects of the Alkaline Diet on the body, the known advantages are significant enough to position the diet as a viable option. If anything, you will substantially enhance your bone health and significantly increase your energy levels.

Chapter 4: Scientific Merit

Dr. Otto Warburg, a German national, was born in the year 1883. It can be speculated that his decision to pursue a career in medicine was influenced by his father, a physicist. During the course of his professional journey, he was honored with numerous accolades in recognition of his comprehensive research on the process of carbon dioxide assimilation in plants and its correlation with tumor formation, encompassing an investigation into the mechanism of oxygen transfer as well. He is frequently regarded as the progenitor of the Alkaline Diet, as his breakthroughs paved the path for numerous advancements in the medical domain that continue to be employed and advanced in the present era.

Following his numerous prior accolades, his most significant accomplishment came in the form of capturing the Nobel Peace Prize in 1931 for his groundbreaking contributions to the field of cancer research. It is worth noting that this esteemed recognition came about after his name had been put forward for consideration a remarkable tally of 46 times. His research has discovered that cancer cells have a sole ability to sustain themselves exclusively in an acidic condition. Conversely, these cells are unable to sustain themselves within an environment abundant in oxygen, such as the balanced pH state of the human body. This is among the factors contributing to the effectiveness of the Alkaline diet in

147

combating cancers and other illnesses. By inducing an alkaline state in the host's body, the proliferation of cancer-causing cells is hindered. The presence of oxygen deficiency was observed within the cancer cells, causing a shift from aerobic metabolism to a less advanced form of respiration characterized by the utilization of sugars present in the body. It was this remarkable finding that precipitated novel advancements in the realms of cellular metabolism and cellular respiration. Therefore, it is critical to acknowledge the adverse requirement of eliminating processed sugars from one's diet, in order to assist in the formation process that does not involve cancer. Dr. Warburg's hypothesis included the belief that the majority of diseases are attributed to pollution, which subsequently results in excessive exposure of the body to toxins. Thus, the merging of these toxins with cells that are malnourished, rich in natural oxygen, and adequately hydrated by sugar constitutes the main etiological factor of cancer. In such instances, the cells develop an inherent defensive mechanism, wherein they utilize sugar fermentation as a means to generate oxygen, allowing for their proliferation while exhibiting resistance to apoptosis. As the progression of cancer takes place, it is the cancer cells themselves that induce a significant increase in acidity within the body.

Dr. Warburg's research revealed that providing cells with sufficient oxygen can inhibit the proliferation of cancer cells, or even induce their gradual demise. The Alkaline Diet plays a crucial role in enhancing the production of oxygen in the bloodstream and significantly diminishing the availability of fermented sugars that cancer cells thrive on, thus occasionally leading to reversal of their growth.

Dr. Warburg authored numerous publications and held the esteemed position of foreign member in the Royal Society of London. In addition, he was bestowed with an honorary doctorate from Oxford University.

Until the passing of Dr. Warburg in 1970, he continued to engage in the pursuit of scholarship and investigation, albeit in a reduced capacity as he collaborated with Dr. Carl Reich on a part-time basis. In this setting, they were conducting conclusive experiments pertaining to cancer, the outcomes of which would have culminated in the publication of a comprehensive research document showcasing their discoveries that had profound implications for the revolutionizing of cancer treatment. According to reports, following the demise of Dr. Reich, it has been noted that he encountered challenges in retrieving his personal apparatus utilized in their scientific investigations, as well as the entirety of their amassed research.

Furthermore, it was ascertained that these findings had yet to be made available to the general population.

Several of Dr. Warburg's subsequent discoveries pertained to the insufficient presence of enzymes in prepared dishes, leading to the aggregation of red blood cells. Once these foods experience an enzyme deficiency, their ability to traverse narrower veins is compromised, thereby giving rise to circulatory complications in various regions of the body. Furthermore, it is within these anatomical regions that possess restricted or negligible oxygen levels that the formation of cancer occurs. However, once an individual attains a stable alkaline condition, there should be no grounds for the accumulation of blood cells in these areas, as the blood cells will be adequately oxygenated and able to circulate unrestrictedly. Now, one can discern the significance of maintaining a balanced body pH level through the incorporation of green vegetables, legumes, and appropriate quantities of nutritious fruits in one's dietary regimen. The objective is to compel the cells, which previously relied on sugars for nourishment, to now rely on oxygen for respiration. If you are experiencing any physical conditions, health issues, or diseases, including those that may be undiagnosed, it is possible to treat or reverse them before they progress to the stage where non-oxygenated cells can facilitate the development of cancer. As per the clinical studies conducted by Warburg.

The accomplishments of a single individual are difficult to fathom, as throughout the majority of his professional trajectory, he has spearheaded numerous concepts and advancements within the realm of the medical sector. Furthermore, had it not been for him, it might have taken another century for someone to establish the connection between the fragments. Additionally, the

Alkaline Diet offers a myriad of advantages and the potential to address previously deemed incurable ailments, traditionally requiring pharmaceutical intervention or chemotherapy. These benefits may be achieved effortlessly through the enhancement and diligent upkeep of one's dietary practices.

An overwhelming majority of illnesses and diseases are not attributed to natural phenomena, but rather stem from human activities. The consistent and prolonged exposure to heavily processed substances and toxins that pervade our daily existence gradually tilts our bodies towards an unstable acidic state, over an extended period of time.

Ultimately, the remedies required to address your illness or disease can be achieved through the collaboration of the nourishing elements of nature and your personal efforts. For this very rationale, it is with utmost gratitude that I express my appreciation to Dr. Otto Warburg, acknowledging his invaluable contributions, albeit posthumously, and recognizing the profound sense of satisfaction and joy he would have derived from witnessing the remarkable accomplishments and positive impact realized by those he had tirelessly supported. We extend our deepest gratitude to Dr. Warburg for his exceptional contributions to the advancement of the human cause; we pay tribute to his exemplary achievements.

www.ingramcontent.com/pod-product-compliance
Lightning Source LLC
Chambersburg PA
CBHW051736020426
42333CB00014B/1330